NINJA FOODI AIR FRYER AND PRESSURE COOKER COOKBOOK

30 COMPLETE QUICK AND DELICIOUS RECIPES FOR BOTH INDOOR AND OUTDOOR GRILLING AND AIR FRYINGS FOR BEGINNERS AND EXPERTS

BILL HEMSWORTH

Copyright

Disclaimer Notice:

Note that it is important that the following information contained in this book is for educational purposes only. After carrying out enough research work, we present a piece of detailed and accurate information as it relates to the present norm. We got the contents in this book from various sources, and hence, the intending readers are not given a warranty. We advise readers to talk to their licensed doctors before trying out the techniques given within this book.

By consenting to this document, the reader accepts that the author is not responsible for any loss either directly or indirectly that can be incurred as a result of the information contained within this book, and also the omissions, errors, or inadequacies of the reader.

Dedication

I dedicate this book to all cooks. In our homes today, as always, life is centered around the kitchen. Some of the recipes I have complied are treasured family keepsakes and some are new; however, they all reflect the love of good cooking.

I hope you all enjoy the many outstanding and treasured recipes on the pages that follow.

Table of content

Introduction

Ninja Foodi is a Pressure Cooker & Air Fryer that can be used as an oven, steamer, roaster, dehydrator, and slow cooker. It makes quick and easily produce delicious snacks, meals, sides & desserts in one particular pot. Tender Crisp Technology speedily cooks to lock in juices, then crisps for a golden finish. Cook mains & sides at the same time, even from frozen. Keep Warm feature. Dishwasher-safe parts. It is easy to operate. It works similarly to the instant pot and other electric pressure cookers.

Cooks & crisps. Pressure cook to start. At that point, switch lids for the perfect finish. Tender Crisp Technology rapidly cooks to lock in juices, then provides your flawlessly cooked food a golden finish with the use of Air Crisp, Grill, or roast settings – from crispy chicken wings to delicious salmon, chunky chips to roasted vegetable, the options are limitless.

These settings are also included: stir fry, steam, grill, fry, slow cook, boil, fast stew, braise.

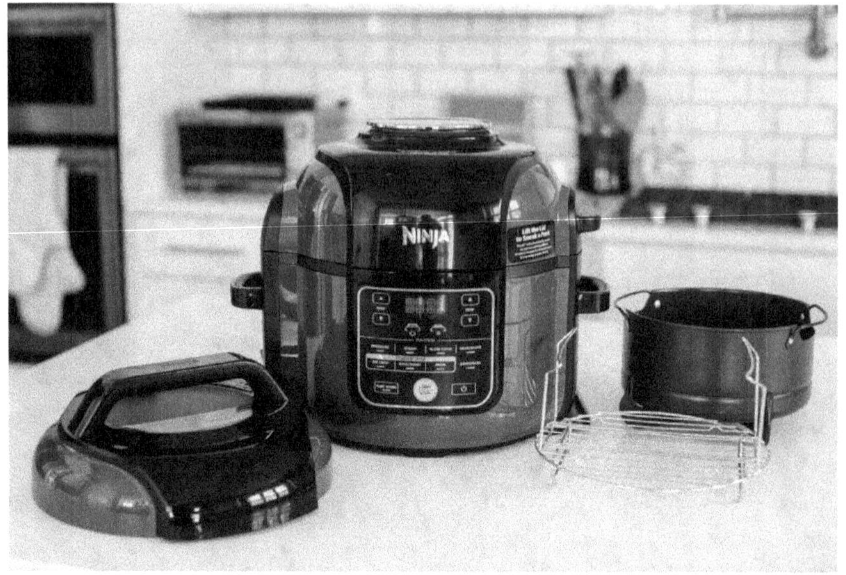

This book will guide you through how to prepare 30 great meals with Ninja Foodi Air fryer and pressure cooker.

EASY AIR FRYER ONION RINGS RECIPE

Ingredients

1. One cup of buttermilk.

2. Two beaten eggs.

3. Salt

4. One large white onion (sliced about ¼ inch slices).

5. Two cups of Gluten-Free all-purpose or regular flour

6. Two cups of regular bread crumbs or Gluten-free breadcrumbs.

Procedures

1. Gently place the onions in a clean, shallow bowl and pour the buttermilk all over them.

2. Allow them to sit and soak for one to two hours.

3. Organize a clean bowl for the flour, a separate bowl for breadcrumbs, and another bowl for the beaten eggs.

4. Apply a dash of salt to the breadcrumbs.

5. Gently dip the onions in the flour and dust off any excess.

6. Gently dip them in the eggs and let the excess drip off.

7. Coat with breadcrumbs,

8. Carefully place evenly in the air fryer.

9. You can proceed to add salt after they are done or before.

10. Fry them in the air fryer for about five minutes at 390 degrees on each side until they are crispy.

11. Spray with cooking spray to get them to become brown in color if you prefer it.

Then serve!

HONEY MUSTARD PORK CHOPS

Equipment

1. Meat thermometer

2. Ninja air fryer

3. Silicone tongs

Recipes

1. One tablespoon of ground black pepper

2. One teaspoon of kosher salt

3. Two tablespoons of honey

4. Two tablespoons of minced garlic

5. Four tablespoons of prepared mustard

6. Four pork chops

7. Cooking oil spray

Procedures

1. Mix together the honey, mustard, salt, pepper, and garlic in a large bowl.

2. Then add the pork chops and gently toss to coat with the sauce you made.

3. Gently spray the air fryer basket. Then place the chops inside the greased basket.

4. Kindly set the air fryer to 350°F until the pork is cooked through, turning upside down halfway through and spraying again with oil.

5. Ensure to flip the chops and keep spraying with oil again halfway through the process of cooking.

6. Avoid piling the chops when cooking them. Ensure there is enough room for the hot air to circulate well and cook the chops.

CRISPY BACON IN AN AIR FRYER

To prepare this meal, all you need is your air fryer and the bacon. This procedure is so simple and easy.

Ingredients

1. One pound of bacon

Procedures

1. Gently add bacon into the air fryer basket. This may take up to two batches to cook all the bacon depending on the size of the bacon.
2. Cook for five minutes at 350 degrees.
3. Gently turn bacon and keep cooking for additional five minutes till you get your desired bacon crispiness.
4. Slowly remove bacon with tongs and place it on a paper towel-lined plate.

Allow to cool, serve, and enjoy!

AIR FRYER HONEY GARLIC SHRIMP

Ingredients:

1. One teaspoon of fresh ginger

2. One clove of crushed garlic

3. Two tablespoons of cornstarch

4. Half cup of honey

5. Half cup of Tamari Gluten Free Soy Sauce

6. Two tablespoons of Ketchup

7. Sixteen ounces of frozen mixed stir-fry vegetable blend.

8. Sixteen ounces of medium fresh shrimp, peeled and deveined.

9. Cooked rice(optional)

Procedures

1. Add together the soy sauce, garlic, ginger, Ketchup, and all the honey in a medium-sized saucepan.

2. Allow to warm up to a low-boil state, then whisk in the cornstarch until the sauce is thickened.

3. Gently coat the shrimp with the sauce.

4. Then line the air fryer with foil, and proceed to add in the shrimp and vegetables.

5. Cook for ten minutes at 355 degrees.

Proceed and serve over cooked rice.

CAJUN SHRIMP BOIL IN THE AIR FRYER

Ingredients

1. Olive oil spray

2. Four mini corn on the cobs

3. Fourteen ounces of sliced smoked sausage rope.

4. Four cups of halved par-boiled small potatoes.

5. Twelve ounces of medium shrimp, peeled and deveined with tail-on (cooked and frozen shrimp)

6. A quarter cup of diced white onion.

7. 1/8 cup of old bay seasoning.

Procedures

1. Kindly par-boil the potatoes. And make use of small potatoes, you can cut in half for this particular recipe.

2. Then combine the remaining ingredients into a very clean large bowl and mix very well once the potatoes are done.

3. Gently place a sheet of foil into the air fryer, make certain that air is still able to circulate.

4. Then add in half of the mixture on top of the foil to fill in the air fryer basket.

5. After adding the ingredients, proceed to spray with a nice coat of olive oil.

6. Cook for six minutes at 390 degrees.

7. Then open the air fryer and carefully mix the ingredients.

8. Cook for an extra six minutes.

9. You can repeat these steps for the next cooking batch if needed.

Cool, serve, and enjoy!

Notes

Kindly note that almost every air fryer heats differently. The air fryer I made use of does not need to be pre-heated. If yours does, be certain to pre-heat and then proceed with the procedures.

After twelve minutes, it ought to be well cooked and warm. Furthermore, entirely all air fryers heat in a different way, so just be certain it's warmed up to your favorite. I constantly commend close inspection of the dish halfway through the cooking time to be sure it's cooking nice and calmly.

20 MINUTE AIR FRYER CHICKEN WINGS (NINJA FOODI)

Ingredients

1. Salt

2. Pepper

3. Barbecue sauce

4. Olive oil spray

5. Six to twelve pieces of chicken wings (Drumettes and Flat)

Procedures

1. Gently spray the foil-lined air fryer basket or air fryer basket with non-stick cooking spray.

2. Carefully place the wings into the basket. In a four-quart air fryer basket, six wings will fit perfectly well.

3. Adjust this as mandatory for the size of your air fryer.

4. Add a coat of olive oil spray evenly.

5. Add a dash of pepper & salt to the wings.

6. Cook for ten minutes at 390 degrees

7. Cook and turn for extra ten minutes at the same temperature.

8. The internal temperature of the wings could be at least 165 degrees.

9. If you prefer barbecue sauce, you can coat with it or other dipping sauces.

Notes

Kindly note that each air fryer heats in a different way; mine does not need to be pre-heated before usage. If yours does, gently pre-heat as ordinary and then proceed with the process of cooking the wings.

AIR FRYER RANCH BREADED PORK CHOPS

Ingredients

1. One package ranch of seasoning mix

2. Two beaten eggs

3. Four boneless thin pork chops

4. Quarter cup bread crumbs, alternatively gluten-free bread crumbs

Procedures

1. Gently place the beaten eggs in a clean bowl.

2. Then mix together the seasoning mix and the bread crumbs in a different bowl.

3. Proceed to dip the pork chops in the eggs and shake off the excess remains.

4. Care spray the basket with a non-stick cooking spray, alternatively line it with foil, and gently spray

the foil. Kindly dip in the seasoning mixture and gently place it in the sprayed air fryer basket.

5. Cook for four minutes at 360 degrees

6. Turn the pork chops and cook it for extra four minutes.

7. If you prefer lightly spray, you can make use of olive oil for spraying.

8. One hundred forty-five degrees is the needed degrees for pork chops to be fully cooked.

Then serve and enjoy!

Notes

It's very vital to note that for this kind of recipe, I made use of tinny cut pork chops. If you make use of thick-cut pork chops or center-cut or thick-cut pork chops, the estimated cooking time will be twelve minutes.

AIR FRYER SHRIMP AND VEGETABLES

Ingredients

1. Cooked rice

2. Olive oil spray

3. One bag of frozen mixed vegetables

4. One tablespoon of Gluten-free cajun seasoning

5. Raw peeled and deveined small shrimp (Regular sized bag about 45-80 small shrimp)

Procedures

1. Add the vegetable and shrimps to your air fryer.

2. Gently top it up with cajun seasoning and apply spray with an even coat of spray.

3. Cook for ten minutes at 355 degrees

4. Gently open and mix up the vegetables and shrimps.

5. Keep cooking for additional ten minutes at 355 degrees.

Cool, serve, and enjoy!

GLUTEN-FREE AIR FRYER CHICKEN FRIED RICE

Ingredients

1. Coconut oil cooking spray.

2. A cup of fully cooked & Diced Chicken Breast.

3. Four to six tablespoons of soy sauce or

4. Four to six Gluten-Free soy sauce

5. Four cups of cold cooked white rice.

6. ¼ cup of diced carrots.

7. ¼ cup of diced celery.

8. ¼ cup of white diced onion.

Procedures

1. Carefully line the air fryer with foil. Make sure the entire basket is not covered to ensure air is able to flow. It's best to roll it up on the side.

2. Gently spray the foil with coconut oil spray.

3. Add up all the ingredients in order on top of the foil in the basket.

4. Mix together by stirring and add a nice coat of coconut oil spray to the top of the mixture.

5. Gently cook in the air fryer at 390 degrees for five minutes.

6. Gently open and stir up the mixture again.

7. Add up an extra coat of spray or soy if it's needed.

8. Keep cooking at 390 degrees for additional five minutes.

Cool, stir, and enjoy!

Notes

A friendly reminder that many times air fryers work in a different way, so if needed, you can add a little bit longer or shorter cooking time. Checking it at five minutes will help you determine if yours needs to cook an additional five minutes.

A cooked and beaten egg is also a nice mixing for this Air Fryer Chicken Fried Rice.

AIR FRYER HONEY GARLIC CHICKEN

Ingredients

1. Green sliced onions.

2. Cooked rice

3. Cornstarch or potato starch

4. Cooked green beans

5. One tablespoon of Cornstarch

6. Six boneless, skinless chicken thighs

7. Half cup of honey

8. Two tablespoons of brown sugar

9. Two tablespoons of Ketchup.

10. One clove of crushed garlic.

11. Half tablespoon of Ground Ginger

12. Half cup of soy sauce or Gluten Free Soy Sauce

13. One clove of crushed garlic.

Procedures

1. Gently cut the chicken into cubelike chunks; after that, toss in a bowl with Potato starch or cornstarch.

2. Make use of sufficient to coat the chicken calmly.

3. Carefully place in the air fryer and continue cooking according to your Air Fryer Manual for Chicken.

4. Combine the honey, brown sugar, Ketchup, ginger, garlic, and Soy Sauce in a small Saucepan while the chicken is cooking.

5. Tune to a low boil, keep whisking in the cornstarch until sauce is thickened. If it's not thick enough, then you can add in additional cornstarch until nicely thickened.

6. Carefully set aside.

7. Once the chicken is fully cooked, gently mix it into the sauce and warm it up.

8. This can be achieved in a small saucepan; just coat the chicken with the sauce because it can be a sticky texture sauce.

9. Cool and serve the chicken on top of the cooked rice with green beans.

Proceed to garnish with green onion.

Notes

If you are producing this in the Ninja Foodi

When you have the chicken readily made, carefully remove the basket. It will tend to be hot; make use of oven mitts. Make sure the pot is properly cleaned out, then you can do your sauce in this particular pot. Basically, make use of the sauté function on medium-high heat.

Kindly make certain to make use of a wooden utensil or one that won't scratch the body of the pot. Stir it very well until it's well combined, then carefully mix in the chicken.

The rice and green beans may also be made in this procedure; however, I find it faster to do it on the stove whilst the chicken is still cooking. That should be your preference.

VEGAN SHEPHERD'S PIE

Ingredients

1. 1/8 cup of Almond milk or coconut milk.

2. Eight medium baking potatoes.

3. One tablespoon of vegan butter and vegan flour.

4. Salt and pepper.

5. Four cups of Vegetable Broth.

6. Two tablespoons of Ketchup.

7. One tablespoon of Garlic Powder.

8. One tablespoon of Rosemary

9. Three cups of mixed vegetables.

10.   One & a half cup of Brown Lentils Rinsed and Uncooked.

11. Three cups of sliced Portobella Mushrooms.

12. Two tablespoons of Pompeian Organic Extra Virgin Olive Oil.

13. A quarter cup of Diced Onions.

Procedures

1. kickstart by pre-heating the oven to 375 degrees.

2. Then place the potatoes in the clean stockpot, and cover with water and bring to boil; keep boiling until it becomes soft.

3. Gently peel the potatoes and place them in a large clean bowl to mix. Then add in the butter and milk along with the pepper and salt to taste and mix very well.

4. Add up the olive oil to a large stockpot and warm up while the potatoes are cooking.

5. Then add the mushroom and onion, and cook for ten minutes or till it softens.

6. Add up the remaining ingredients and stir to mix well.

7. Allow to warm up to a low boil for about twenty minutes and stir frequently.

8. Carefully spray a 9 x 13 baking dish with a non-stick cooking spray and pour the filling mixture into the dish, and spread calmly.

9. Add potatoes and spread calmly with a fork, and add a dash of Rosemary, pepper, and salt to top. Bake for fifty minutes or till the potatoes is evenly browned.

AIR FRYER PIZZA BAGELS

Ingredients

1. Pizza sauce.

2. Mozzarella cheese

3. One package of Gluten-Free Bagels or plain Bagels.

4. Mini pepperonis, cooked chicken, or sausage.

Procedures

1. Gently cut the bagels in half.

2. Then top each bagel with the sauce and toppings of your desired choice.

3. Carefully coat with cheese.

4. Cook in the air fryer at 355 degrees for five minutes.

Cool, serve, and enjoy!

AIR FRYER DEEP-DISH PEPPERONI PIZZA

Ingredients

1. One cup of shredded mozzarella cheese.

2. Two tablespoons of shredded parmesan cheese.

3. Eleven pepperoni slices.

4. 1/3 cup of pizza sauce.

5. One can of refrigerated classic pizza crust.

6. One tablespoon of olive oil.

Procedures

1. Carefully cut an 8-inch round of cooking parchment paper.

2. Place in the bottom of the air fryer basket.

3. Spray the air fryer basket with cooking spray.

4. Gently unroll dough and tuck corners under.

5. Shape it into a 10-inch round with a 1-inch thicker border.

6. Gently press into air fryer basket on top of parchment then press one and a half inches up side of the basket.

7. Then set to 325 degrees, cook for ten minutes. Turn your pizza crust over on the counter and remove parchment and replace it in the air fryer basket.

8. Cook two to three minutes or till it becomes cool enough to handle.

9. Making use of fingers, press down the center of crust, making a one-inch border. Brush sides and the top of crust all over, making use of olive oil, and place in the basket. Then cook for additional five minutes.

Top the center of the dough with the pizza sauce. Also, top with mozzarella cheese, furthermore top with pepperoni, followed up by Parmesan cheese. Cook for four to seven minutes longer or until properly cooked through and the cheese is melted. Cool it down for two minutes. Then remove from the basket with a rubber spatula.

AIR FRYER SEASONED ASPARAGUS

Ingredients

1. Garlic salt

2. One bunch of Asparagus

3. Cooking spray (Olive oil)

Procedures

1. Commence by trimming up to two inches off the stems of the Asparagus.

2. Then add the Asparagus to the basket of the air fryer.

3. Gently coat with olive oil spray and a little dash of garlic salt.

4. Cook for five minutes at 390 degrees.

5. Inspect the Asparagus and flip it

6. Cook for additional five minutes

Allow cooling, then serve.

AIR FRYER GLAZED CHICKEN THIGHS (NINJA FOODI)

Ingredients

1. Eight Boneless, Skinless Chicken Thighs.

2. One tablespoon of crushed garlic.

3. Two tablespoons of brown sugar.

4. Two tablespoons of Gluten-Free Soy Sauce.

5. One tablespoon of peeled, grated ginger.

6. Half tablespoon of Gluten-free Worcestershire sauce.

Procedures

1. Get a clean small bowl and combine the soy sauce, ginger, garlic, brown sugar, and Worcestershire sauce.

2. Gently place the chicken thighs in a Ziplock bag, then add in the sauce and make sure it coats the chicken completely.

3. Let these sit for up to three hours or more.

4. When it's ready to make, gently cook in the air fryer at 390 degrees for five minutes, then flip and cook for extra five minutes.

5. The temperature should be at a minimum of 165 degrees before serving.

Notes:

Constant check the chicken at five minutes and cook for an extra five minutes on each side of the chicken if needed to reach that internal temperature of 165 degrees. Many times, air fryers all heat in a different way, so the times might need to be adjusted to fit perfectly for yours.

AIR FRYER FRIED PICKLES

Ingredients

1. Two beaten eggs.

2. One cup of buttermilk.

3. Salt

4. Two cups of regular bread crumbs or Gluten-Free breadcrumbs.

5. Two cups of drained sliced pickles.

6. Two cups of regular flour or Gluten-Free all-purpose flour.

Procedures

1. Gently place the pickles in a clean, shallow bowl and pour the buttermilk all over them.

2. Allow them to sit and soak for one to two hours.

3. Organize a clean bowl for the flour, a separate bowl for breadcrumbs, and another bowl for the beaten eggs.

4. Apply a dash of salt to the breadcrumbs.

5. Gently dip the pickles in the flour and dust off any excess.

6. Gently dip them in the eggs and let the excess drip off.

7. Coat with breadcrumbs,

8. Carefully place evenly in the air fryer.

9. You can proceed to add salt after they are done or before.

10. Fry them in the air fryer for about five minutes at 390 degrees on each side until they are crispy.

11. Spray with cooking spray to get them to become brown in color if you prefer it.

Then serve!

TACO STYLE QUINOA STUFFED AVOCADO

Ingredients

1. Four Avocados

2. Two cups of cooked Quinoa

3. One package of Taco seasoning.

4. Pompeian Avocado oil spray.

Toppings

1. Lettuce

2. Tomato

3. Cilantro

4. Bell pepper

5. Shredded cheese

6. Catalina Dressing

7. Sour cream.

Procedures

1. Gently slice the avocados into two halves and remove the seed.

2. Carefully spray each half with Pompeian Avocado Oil Spray.

3. Then place cut side down into a grill which has been warmed to medium-high heat.

4. Continue grilling for five minutes or till it gets toasted.

5. Mix the cooked and warm Quinoa with taco seasoning while this is grilled.

6. Stuff each Avocado with Quinoa and toppings of your preference once the Avocado is done.

Serve and Enjoy!

AIR FRYER GARLIC BREAD PIZZA TOAST

Ingredients

1. One cup of shredded mozzarella cheese.

2. One cup of pizza sauce

3. ½ cup of pepperoni

4. One package of garlic Texas toast

Procedures

1. Carefully place the toast in the basket inside the air fryer.

2. Gently top each piece with pepperoni, cheese, and sauce.

3. Cook for five minutes at 360 degrees.

Cool, serve, and enjoy!

Notes

Kindly remember that you can do this at 355 degrees or slightly higher depending on the choices on your air fryer. This, too, can be modified to your preferred toppings.

PERFECT PERSONAL PIZZAS IN AN AIR FRYER

Ingredients

1. Two tablespoons of jarred pizza sauce.

2. Six or seven mini pepperonis.

3. Two tablespoons of shredded pizza cheese, alternatively shredded mozzarella.

4. One Stonegate of mini naan round

Procedure

1. Gently top the mini naan round with shredded pizza cheese, pizza sauce, and mini pepperoni.

2. Carefully place the topped personal pizza into the clean basket of an air fryer.

3. Then set the air fryer to about 375 degrees.

4. Fry the pizza for like five to seven minutes or until the cheese is completely melted or starting to brown.

Serve and enjoy immediately.

AIR FRYER SAUSAGE, BEANS, & POTATO HASH

Ingredients

1. One teaspoon of no salt added seasoning.

2. One hundred ounces of a frozen bag of green beans.

3. Four cups of potatoes, Quartered.

4. One olive oil spray.

5. One packaged cocktail sausage.

procedures

1. Gently wash and cut the potatoes and place a sheet of foil in the bottom of the air fryer or you can make use of the basket of the air fryer.

2. Gently spray the basket or foil with olive oil spray.

3. Gently place the potatoes on the bottom, top filled with sausages and green beans. The green beans basically do not need to be softened.

4. Add your preferred seasoning and carefully spray with a nice coat of olive oil spray.

5. Cook in the air fryer at 355 degrees for twenty-five minutes.

6. Halt the cooking halfway through, then mix up the ingredients to flip them then avoid burning.

At this stage, you can spray with extra olive oil if needed, remove, then serve!

Notes

Concerning the sausage, I made use of the 14oz Package of Lil' Smokies. There exists a 12oz package that would work perfectly too. The larger amount would also do the work, but it may require to be cooked in two batches depending on the sizes of the Air Fryer.

Concerning foil, if you make use of foil, be certain not to cover the entire bottom of the basket. Ensure that air can still flow through.

Recall that all air fryers work in a different way. I recommend inspecting the food around halfway through cook time and turning it, mixing it up with a clean spoon. Then, proceed with cooking. Every now and then, depending on the air fryer that you may have, it can take a shorter time or longer time to prepare.

EASY AIR FRYER HUSH PUPPIES (NINJA FOODI)

Ingredients

1. One egg

2. ¾ cup of milk

3. ¼ cup of chopped onions.

4. Half teaspoon of salt.

5. One and a half cup of Gluten-free All-purpose flour or All-purpose flour.

6. ¼ teaspoon of sugar.

7. One cup of yellow cornmeal.

8. One & a half teaspoon of Baking powder.

Procedures

1. Combine baking powder, sugar, flour, cornmeal, and salt in a large bowl and mix in the onions.

2. Then whisk in the milk and egg.

3. Let batter sit out for about five minutes.

4. Create small balls of dough to form hush puppies.

5. Gently place them inside the air fryer, you can line the inside of the air fryer with foil, or preferably you can spray the bottom with non-stick cooking spray.

6. Spray them in addition to olive oil or a coat of non-stick cooking spray.

7. Cook in the air fryer for approximately 5 minutes at 390 degrees.

8. Carefully turn them upside down and spray them with the use of olive oil or coat with a non-stick cooking spray for extra five minutes.

Serve and enjoy!

NOTE: serve it when crispy; also, remember that all air fryers put off a different degree of heat. Ensure to check them continue cooking for a few extra minutes if it needs.

AIR FRYER HONEY GARLIC CHICKEN

Ingredients

1. Sliced Green Onions.

2. Cooked green beans and rice.

3. Two tablespoons of Brown sugar and Ketchup

4. Half cup of honey

5. Potato Starch and Cornstarch

6. Six boneless, skinless chicken thighs.

7. ½ cup of Soy Sauce or Gluten-free soy sauce.

8. Half tablespoon of Ground Ginger.

9. One clove of Crushed Garlic.

Procedures

1. Carefully cut the chicken into cubed portions, then toss it in a bowl with potato starch or cornstarch, fmaking use of enough to coat the chicken evenly.

2. Then gently place in the Air Fryer and cook according to your Air Fryer manual for chicken. (while cooking mine, it took me twenty-four minutes, twelve minutes on each side on 390 degrees).

3. While the chicken is still cooking, in a small clean saucepan, combine the soy sauce, honey, garlic, ginger, ketchup, and brown sugar.

4. Set it to a low boil, then paddle in the cornstarch until the sauce becomes thickened. If it's not thick enough, carefully add in extra cornstarch until it becomes thickened.

5. Set it aside, and once the chicken is properly cooked, then mix it into the sauce and warm it up. This can be achieved in a small saucepan. Just coat the chicken with the sauce because it will be a sticky texture sauce.

6. Proceed to serve the chicken over the cooked rice with green beans and garnish with green onions.

If you want to produce this in the Ninja Foodi

As soon as you have the chicken made, cautiously remove the basket. It will be hot, make use of oven mitts. Then clean the pot out, then you can do your sauce in this cleaned pot. Basically, make use of the sauté function on medium-high heat. Ensure to make use of a wooden utensil or one that won't scratch the body of the pot. Stir it until it's well-collected, then mix in all chicken.

The rice and green beans may also be done in this; nevertheless, I discover that it's faster to just do those on the stove despite the fact the chicken is cooking. That's your choice.

AIR FRYER PLATE NACHOS

Ingredients

1. Diced green onions.

2. Tortilla Chips.

3. White Queso.

4. Grilled chicken (cooked)

5. Drained and Rinsed Black Beans.

6. Halved Grape Tomatoes.

Procedures

1. Carefully line the basket of the Air Fryer with foil.

2. Apply non-stick spray.

3. Assemble the nachos, add the chips, beans, and chicken.

4. Add a layer of queso and top with onions and tomatoes.

5. Carefully turn the air fryer to 355 degrees for five minutes, or you can add extra time until your desired level of crispiness is reached.

INSTANT POT HEARTY BEAN CHILI (NINJA FOODI)

Ingredients

1. ½ cup of Ketchup

2. One teaspoon of Chili powder

3. One crushed of garlic clove.

4. Two cups of Chili Beans.

5. One tablespoon of Organic Extra virgin oil.

6. Two cups of diced tomatoes.

7. 14.5 ounces of Can of Beef Broth.

8. One pound of lean Ground beef.

9. ¼ cup of Diced White onion.

10. Two cups of red kidney beans.

Toppings

1. Chives

2. Sour cream

3. Corn chips

4. Cornbread

5. Shredded cheese

6. Parsley

Procedures

1. Place the instant pot on the sauté function.

2. Then add the olive oil to the clean bowl of the instant pot.

3. Add up the ground beef and cook it until it's almost done.

4. Add in the onions and keep cooking until both the ground beef and the onions are done, also. Add in the remaining ingredients.

5. Mix everything together and add a lid to the instant pot to ensure the vent is sealed. And cook for four minutes on high pressure.

Carefully release the steam once it is done, then stir and serve!

VEGAN SHEPHERD'S PIE

Ingredients

1. Salt and pepper to taste.

2. One teaspoon of garlic powder.

3. Two tablespoons of Ketchup.

4. Potatoes.

5. Eight medium of baking potatoes.

6. ¼ cup of diced onion.

7. 1/8 cup of Almond milk or coconut milk.

8. Filling

9. One tablespoon of vegan butter.

10. One tablespoon of vegan flour.

11. Four cups of Vegetable Broth.

12. One and a half cups of rinsed and uncooked brown lentils.

13. One tablespoon of Rosemary.

14. Three cups of mixed vegetables.

15. Two tablespoons of Pompeian organic extra virgin olive oil.

16. Three cups of sliced portobello Mushrooms.

Procedures

1. kickstart the procedure by pre-heating the oven to 375 degrees.

2. Gently place the potatoes in the stockpot and cover with water, and boil.

3. Keep boiling at a low temperature until it becomes soft.

4. Gently peel the potatoes and place them in a large clean bowl to mix.

5. Add butter and milk, along with the pepper and salt, to give good taste and mix well.

6. Add olive oil to a large clean pot and warm up while the potatoes are cooking.

7. Add in the onions and mushroom, continue cooking for ten minutes until it becomes soft.

8. Add the remaining ingredients, stir to combine.

9. Allow to warm up to a low boil for about fifteen minutes and stir occasionally.

10.   Carefully spray a 9 x 13 baking dish with a non-stick cooking spray.

11. Then pour the filling mixture into a clean dish and spread calmly.

12. Add up the potatoes and spread well with the use of a fork.

13. Then add a dash of salt, Rosemary, and pepper to the top.

Bake for approximately fifty minutes or till the potatoes is, to some extent, browned.

EASY VEGAN PEACH CRISP

Ingredients

1. Half cup of brown sugar

2. One teaspoon of ground nutmeg.

3. Eight sliced peaches.

4. Half a cup of water.

5. One teaspoon of Ground Cinnamon

6. One cup of Gluten-free rolled oats and Gluten-free all-purpose flour.

7. A quarter teaspoon of baking powder and baking soda.

8. One teaspoon of ground nutmeg.

9. Half cup of Pompeian smooth extra virgin olive oil and Pompeian Organic Extra Virgin Olive Oil spray.

Procedures

1. kickstart by pre-heating the oven to 350 degrees.

2. Apply baking dish with Pompeian Organic Extra Virgin Olive Oil Spray or Spray a round cast iron dish.

3. Gently place the peaches in the dish and top with the nutmeg and cinnamon, and calmly pour the water on top.

4. In another clean bowl, combine the flour, oats, baking powder, baking soda, brown sugar, and olive oil until it tends to shape like butter like structure.

5. Gently pat it evenly on top of the peaches and add another dash of cinnamon if you are not satisfied with the taste.

6. Continue baking at 350 degrees for forty-five minutes or till it's perfectly browned.

Select your choice of vegan ice cream and serve!

TACO STYLE QUINOA STUFFED AVOCADO

Ingredients

1. Four avocados

2. One package of Taco seasoning

3. Two cups of cooked Quinoa

4. Pompeian Avocado Oil Spray

5. Shredded cheese

6. Sour cream

7. Catalina Dressing

8. Lettuce

9. Tomato, Bell pepper, Cilantro, and Toppings.

Procedures

1. Carefully slice the avocados in half and gently remove the seed.

2. Then spray each half with Pompeian avocado oil spray.

3. Gently place and cut side down onto a grill that has been warmed to medium-high heat.

4. Then grill for five minutes or till it gets toasted.

5. While this is being grilled, go ahead and mix the cooked and slightly warm Quinoa all with the taco seasoning.

6. Once the Avocado is being done, gently stuff each Avocado with the Quinoa and topping of your preference.

Serve and enjoy!

CRISPY BACON IN AN AIR FRYER

Ingredients

1. One pound of bacon

Procedure

1. Add the bacon into the air fryer basket calmly. Depending on the size, this may take two batches to finish preparing all of the bacon.

2. Cook for five minutes at 350 degrees.

3. Turn the bacon and cook for additional five minutes or until your favored crispiness is met.

4. Gently remove the bacon with tongs and place them on a clean paper towel-lined plate.

Allow cooling, then serve.

AIR FRYER KOREAN BBQ BEEF

Ingredients

For meat:

1. Pompeian oils coconut spray.

2. ¼ cup of corn starch.

3. One pound of thinly sliced steak or flank steak.

For sauce:

1. One tablespoon of water.

2. One tablespoon of cornstarch

3. One tablespoon of ginger.

4. One crushed clove Garlic

5. Two tablespoons of Pompeian white wine vinegar.

6. ½ cup of brown sugar.

7. ½ cup of soy sauce.

8. ½ tablespoon of sesame seeds.

9. One teaspoon of Hot Chili Sauce.

Procedures

1. Kickstart by preparing the steak first, then thinly slice it and put it in the cornstarch.

2. Line the foil in the air fryer or spray the basket with coconut oil spray.

3. Then add the steak and spray another coat of spray on top of it.

4. Cook in the air fryer for ten minutes at 390 degrees, flip the steak and keep cooking for extra ten minutes.

5. Whilst the steak s still cooking, add up the sauce ingredients, excluding the cornstarch and water, to a medium saucepan.

6. Then warm it up to a low-boil, whisk in the water and cornstarch.

7. Gently remove the steak and pour the sauce over the steak and mix well.

8. Go ahead and serve topped with sliced green onions,
   cooked rice with green beans.

AIR FRYER STUFFED PEPPERS

Ingredients

1. ¼ cup of shredded Mozzarella cheese.

2. One cup of marinara sauce and one cup of cooked rice.

3. Half teaspoon of garlic salt.

4. One pound of lean ground beef.

5. Six green bell peppers.

6. ¼ cup of diced green onion.

7. ½ teaspoon of ground sage.

8. One tablespoon of olive oil

9. ¼ cup of fresh parsley.

Procedures

1. Start by warming up a medium-sized skillet with the ground beef and cook until it is done.

2. Drain beef and revert back to the pan and add the olive oil, parsley, green onion, salt, and sage, also add in the cooked rice and marinara, and mix well.

3. Gently cut the top off of each pepper and clean the seeds out very well.

4. Carefully scoop the mixture into each of the peppers and place well in the basket of the air fryer.

5. Cook at 355 degrees for ten minutes in the air fryer function and carefully open and add up cheese.

6. Cook for extra five minutes or until the peppers are slightly soft and cheese is melted.

Allow to cool and serve!

Conclusion

I advise you to inspect the food around halfway through cook time and turn and mix it up with a clean spoon since all air fryers and pressure cookers work in a different way. Determined by the model of air fryer that you may have; it can take a shorter time or longer time to prepare.

Ninja recommends a short trial run with a pot of water if it's your first time using the Ninja Foodi to see how it's done & relax any nerves about exploiting it. As for safety procedures, the lid of the Foodi will never unlock up until pressure is fully released, and there are obvious labels inside the cooking pot to mark the maximum point to where you can add your ingredients; Enjoy!

www.ingramcontent.com/pod-product-compliance
Lightning Source LLC
Chambersburg PA
CBHW061515250726

48657CB00005B/1878